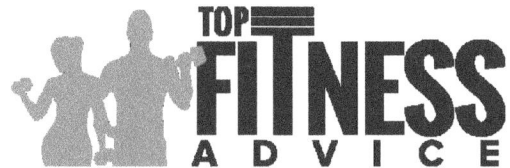

LOSE YOUR BELLY DIET

12 Steps To Blast Belly Fat & Live A Healthier Life!

(BONUS: 30 Healthy & Delicious Food Tips Included)

Kayla Bates

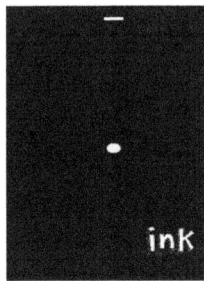

First published in 2017 by Venture Ink Publishing

Copyright © Top Fitness Advice 2019

All rights reserved.

No part of this book may be reproduced in any form without permission in writing from the author. No part of this publication may be reproduced or transmitted in any form or by any means, mechanic, electronic, photocopying, recording, by any storage or retrieval system, or transmitted by email without the permission in writing from the author and publisher.

Requests to the publisher for permission should be addressed to publishing@ventureink.co

For more information about the contents of this book or questions to the author, please contact Kayla Bates at kayla@topfitnessadvice.com

Disclaimer

This book provides wellness management information in an informative and educational manner only, with information that is general in nature and that is not specific to you, the reader. The contents of this book are intended to assist you and other readers in your personal wellness efforts. Consult your physician regarding the applicability of any information provided in this book to you.

Nothing in this book should be construed as personal advice or diagnosis, and must not be used in this manner. The information provided about conditions is general in nature. This information does not cover all possible uses, actions, precautions, side-effects, or interactions of medicines, or medical procedures. The information in this book should not be considered as complete and does not cover all diseases, ailments, physical conditions, or their treatment.

You should consult with your physician before beginning any exercise, weight loss, or health care program. This book should not be used in place of a call or visit to a competent health-care professional. You should consult a health care professional before adopting any of the suggestions in this book or before drawing inferences from it.

Any decision regarding treatment and medication for your condition should be made with the advice and consultation of a qualified health care professional. If you have, or suspect you have, a health-care problem, then you should immediately contact a qualified health care professional for treatment.

No Warranties: The author and publisher don't guarantee or warrant the quality, accuracy, completeness, timeliness, appropriateness or suitability of the information in this book, or of any product or services referenced in this book.

The information in this book is provided on an "as is" basis and the author and publisher make no representations or warranties of any kind with respect to this information. This book may contain inaccuracies, typographical errors, or other errors.

Liability Disclaimer: The publisher, author, and other parties involved in the creation, production, provision of information, or delivery of this book specifically disclaim any responsibility, and shall not be held liable for any damages, claims, injuries, losses, liabilities, costs, or obligations including any direct, indirect, special, incidental, or consequences damages (collectively known as "Damages") whatsoever and howsoever caused, arising out of, or in connection with the use or misuse of the site and the information contained within it, whether such Damages arise in contract, tort, negligence, equity, statute law, or by way of other legal theory.

Table of Contents

Disclaimer	3
Who is this book for?	9
What will this book teach you?	11
Introduction	13
Step 1: Know What You Have to Lose	19
Step 2: Eliminate that Sugar	21
Step 3: Reduce Those Carbs	25
Step 4: Increase Your Soluble Fiber	31
Step 5: Cut Back on the Alcohol Consumption	35
Step 6: Boost the Protein	39
Step 7: Look at Your Stress Levels	45
Step 8: Get the Cardio Workouts Started	49
Step 9: Lift Weights in Your Routine	55
Step 10: Get into a Better Routine	59
Step 11: Watch What You Drink	63
Step 12: Keep Track of Things	65
Conclusion	67

30 Bonus Food Tips   73

Final Words   95

Would you prefer to listen to my book, rather than read it?

Download the audiobook version for free!

If you go to the special link below and sign up to Audible as a new customer, you can get the audiobook version of my book completely free.

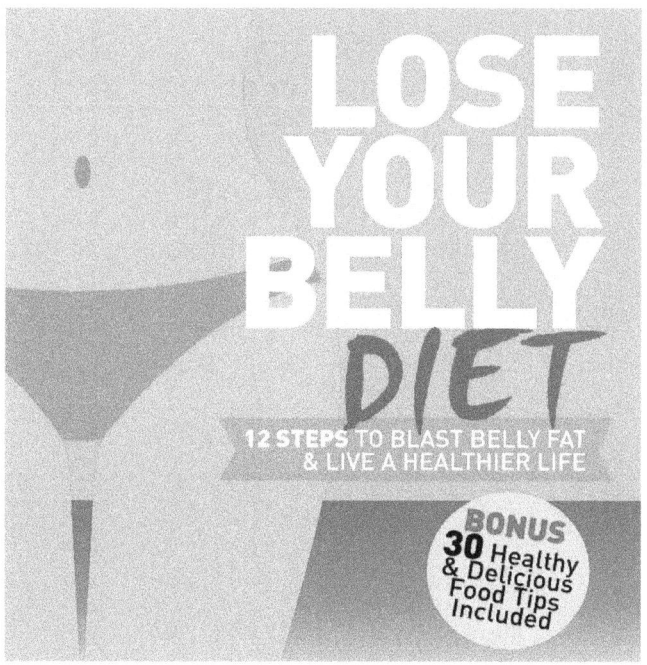

Go here to get your audiobook version for free:

TopFitnessAdvice.com/go/LoseBelly

Who is this book for?

This book is aimed at any individual who is fed up of having that belly fat that just seems to be resistant to all other attempts to remove it.

This alone is stressful and leads to all kinds of negative thoughts and feelings about your appearance, and it's not helped by the fact that it is the hardest part of fat to lose in your entire body.

The aim is to provide the individual with a total of 12 simple steps that can be applied at any point, and that have been shown to be effective at combating the issue of belly fat.

The book also includes 30 ideas for meals that you may wish to incorporate into your diet to not only provide you with all of your nutritional requirements, but also when being kind to your belly.

What will this book teach you?

This book is going to teach you not only how to lose that belly fat, but also better explain the reasons as to why it is such an issue for most people.

It will go into details of the role that sugar and carbs play in all of this.

It will look at diet, the role that stress plays, alcohol, how to work out, and the correct way of doing so.

The book will also educate you on the way in which you can counteract those natural processes in your body to make it easier for you to first of all prevent your body from adding more fat to your belly before you then fight back.

Yes, you will need to understand how to stop putting on weight before you can lose it, and by the end of this book, that is one thing that you will feel far more confident about.

In other words, this book will change your life. It will provide you with the desire and determination to once and for all fight against that belly fat and to stop it from ruining your life. It is going to be tough, but it will all be worth it in the end.

Introduction

Let's face it, is there anything more annoying than trying to lose that belly fat?

It just seems that you can shed that fat on any other part of your body, and yet your belly just wants to hold onto it for as long as possible.

For most people, this ends up being a complete and utter mystery. Just think of the rather confused looks that appear on your face when you look in the mirror and are just bemused as to how that little pouch is still hanging on in there for grim death.

The truth is simple.

You are tackling things in the wrong way.

Now, this is not exactly going to be ground-breaking to hear. After all, you will have probably sassed that out already, but then it opens up another problem.

How exactly do you go ahead and move this stubborn fat?

Well, things can be easier than you may have perhaps initially thought. You will learn this by just following these 12 steps that will not only help you to lose that belly fat, but also help you to go on and live a much happier life as well.

Sound good?

If so, then we really need to get started so you can then start to see a difference around your middle.

But before that, we need to put across some warnings, but there's no need for you to be concerned and getting stressed out (we will tell you why we don't want you to get stressed out later).

Shedding belly fat is important for the sake of your overall health, and not just on the scales. This is known as visceral fat, and it is going to increase your chances of developing Type 2 diabetes and even some heart conditions.

In other words, your health is at risk if you fail to tackle this belly fat issue that you are having, but then you would like to think that your body wouldn't make it so difficult to get rid of it.

Sadly, it does, but then let's get stuck into the 12 steps and see about helping you to remove some of that belly fat as quickly as possible.

Are You ALWAYS Hungry When You Try to Lose Weight?

Discover How to STOP Starving Yourself & Lose Weight FASTER By Eating MORE Food!

For this month only, you can get Kayla's best-selling & most popular book absolutely free – *The Ultimate Guide to Healthy Eating & Losing Weight Without Starving Yourself!*

Get Your FREE Copy Here:
TopFitnessAdvice.com/Book

Discover how you can **start eating MORE food** and see weight loss results faster than ever before. Learn about the 10 most powerful fat-burning foods and how they boost the rate that your body burns fat. And last but not least, finally put an end to your emotional or "bored" eating habits. With this book, readers were able to significantly improve their weight loss results. So, it's highly recommended that you get this book, especially while it's free!

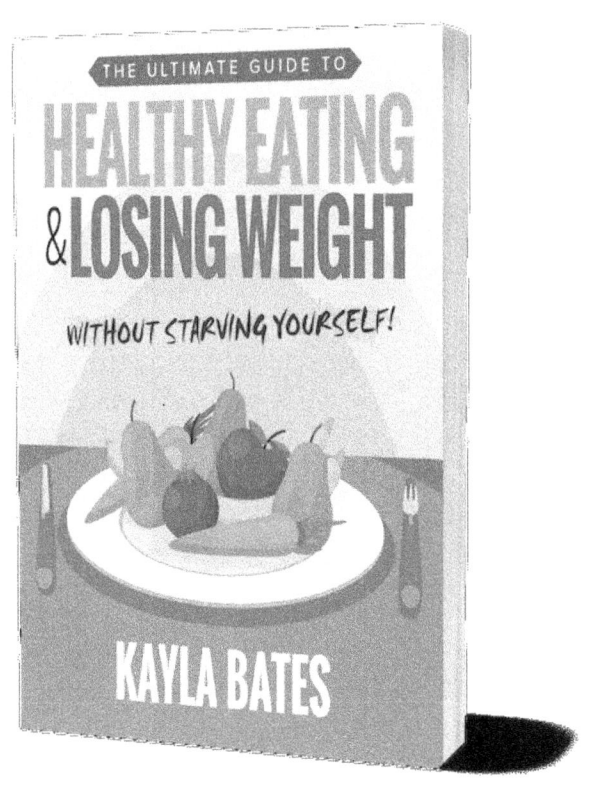

Get Your FREE Copy Here:

TopFitnessAdvice.com/Book

Step 1

Know What You Have to Lose

This is important, but you clearly need to know what it is that you have to lose so you can then establish your targets. Without this, you are attempting to shed some pounds and belly fat when there may not even be any need.

However, there are some very important statistics that you need to be aware of when it comes to knowing what to lose around your middle, and it is connected to the size and what is regarded as being healthy.

As you would expect, there are different measurements for men and women, so this is also something that needs to be taken into consideration.

The problem here is that most people believe that they need to lose more than what is actually required.

They have a completely false sense of reality, and this will then lead to them developing a complex whereby they enter into a depression that they are just not getting rid of that pouch that is perhaps still there.

However, there has to be a realization that, at times, we just have that little last bit that is more difficult to lose than others. It is just the way that we are built.

Some people have a larger middle than others just by nature.

Other people lose weight without putting too much effort in thanks to their metabolism and the general way in which their body reacts.

Step 2

Eliminate that Sugar

A lot of people have a sweet tooth, and if that sounds like you then you have a tough problem to try to overcome.

The problem that you are facing is that sugar is converted into glucose in your body and when it's not being used for energy; it is then being turned into fat. Now, guess where your body decides that it's going to store that fat?

Yep, you guessed right, it's around your belly.

There's no point in going into all of the science behind this and the reasons as to why this is the case. Instead, the most important thing of all is just being aware that sugar is one of the major causes for belly fat to form in the first place.

Of course, cutting out those sugary drinks and candy is going to be easy, but sugar is in so many things that it's impossible to completely cut it out without just eating vegetables.

You need to remember that even fruit is high in naturally occurring sugars, but they can still eventually be converted into fat and stored around your belly.

The Role Sugar Plays in Belly Fat

Just prior to looking more closely at the types of foods that you need to be aware of thanks to the sugar content, it is useful to examine the role that sugar does indeed play in the development of belly fat.

We mentioned it briefly earlier on, but there is slightly more to it.

Sugar is made up of two parts, glucose and fructose. The fructose is an issue as the only part of our body that can really break it down is the liver, but even that has its limitations.

The problem is that this fructose is metabolized by your liver, and in doing so it turns it into fat that is then put into your bloodstream. Your body has no option but to then put this somewhere, as it can then burn it off later as it is in this fat form, and it heads straight to your belly.

But there is another problem that is being caused by fructose, and that is insulin resistance.

Let's get into some basic biology here. The level of glucose that we have in our blood is monitored by our insulin.

If we eat a lot of sugar, then our blood glucose levels will rise as a result, but too much glucose is actually toxic to our body. This then leads to insulin being released which tells our cells to use some of the glucose to reduce the levels of it that's in our blood.

Pretty clever stuff you have to agree. But insulin can also pose its very own problem. It sends out signals to our fat cells whereby it instructs them to pick up fat that's in our bloodstream and to use that rather than the fat that it has already accumulated.

Now, you might think that this is a good thing and, to a certain extent, it is. However, the main problem is that this is the cause of you finding it difficult to move that belly fat.

So, this is what's going on.

You eat a lot of sugar and the levels of fructose are increased, as are the levels of glucose. The fructose is turned into fat and heads to your belly.

The glucose triggers an insulin response, but too much fructose causes issues with your insulin production. It then stops you from burning off the belly fat that you have just put on with the result being you running into all kinds of difficulties in moving that abdominal fat.

Your Steps to Complete this Change

To really take advantage of this step, you simply need to look at your sugar intake and to be aware of how you can go about reducing it on a daily basis. This is not easy, as you will surely testify, but the chances of you losing that belly fat without lowering your sugar intake are non-existent.

Cut out those sugary drinks. Watch how much fruit you eat on a daily basis thanks to the high levels of fructose that appears in it naturally, and don't be fooled into thinking that this is the healthier option as that is not always the case.

Step 3

Reduce Those Carbs

We need carbs, they play a vital role in our diet and completely eliminating them will only lead to you developing various other problems at some point in the future. However, that's not what we are telling you to do.

Instead, our advice is to spend some time reducing the amount of carbs that you are consuming on a daily basis as this will have a profound impact on your ability to shed that belly fat.

Why does this help? Simply because, as with sugar, your body is going to store the carbs that it's not converting into energy around your middle.

However, there is often some confusion with carbs. The confusion is that some people believe that they should be completely removed from your diet, when in actual fact, it has been shown that focusing on removing refined carbs only will be beneficial.

Studies have shown time and time again that refined carbs will help to add that fat to your middle, so it makes sense that removing them from your diet should then have the opposite effect.

But here is something that is quite interesting. If you swap those refined carbs for what is known as unprocessed starchy carbohydrates, or complex carbs as they are otherwise known, then you could still lose belly fat even though carbs are in your diet.

The reason for this is pretty straightforward. Refined carbs are bad for you, but unprocessed complex carbs are good for you, although still in relatively small quantities.

But how is this so? To explain it, we need to look at the actual difference between the two types of carbs as it will then become clear.

The Difference Between Refined Carbs and Complex Carbs

The difference between the two is like day and night. Refined carbs are best explained as being white pasta, white rice, white flour, white anything to be honest. The reason why it is bad is simply because of the way in which the wheat has been processed.

Basically, with a refined carbohydrate, we are looking at something that has been processed by man. The problem with this is that there is a tendency to strip away so much of the goodness that appears in the external kernel of the wheat or cereal and it just leaves the complex sugar chains inside.

If your body is not getting the goodness from it, and is only getting sugar, then you can start to see why this is bad for that abdominal fat.

Complex carbs are, as you may have guessed, wholegrains and items that have not been processed or altered. This means that it also includes starchy vegetables, grains, beans, legumes, anything that is natural and is largely kept in that state.

The reason why this is so good for us is because of the natural fiber content.

This natural fiber is going to be removed when it is being turned into white flour or whatever it may be, so your body is programmed to look for the fiber, and then it is confused when it's not there. It treats those white ingredients as if it is just sugar, which goes straight onto your belly.

Why is it Good for Belly Fat to Eat Complex Carbs?

To best understand why this is so good for belly fat, we need to look at some simple chemistry.

We said earlier how unrefined and complex carbs have a higher fiber content, and that is important. These good carbs take longer to be absorbed into our body, so we are going to feel fuller for longer than before.

Also, as our body takes its time to break it down into its individual components, we avoid getting that spike in our blood sugar level, which then kick starts its own chemical chain that ultimately results in an increase in belly fat.

Basically, you eat refined carbs and your body takes the sugar, as that is the only thing that remains, it triggers the insulin response in your body, the sugar is turned into glucose, and then our body keeps it as there's just too much sugar for it to deal with.

Now, compare that to the other alternative. You eat unrefined carbs. Your body has to take its time breaking down those external aspects. The complex sugar chains that form the core of the carbohydrate takes longer to be broken down.

It enters your blood stream piece by piece rather than all at once. This will then allow your body to deal with the sugar as it goes into your body.

This, in turn, is easier for your body to cope with and it's not going to then trigger the same insulin response leading to that conversion into glucose and fat.

Your Steps to Change Things

In order to actually complete this step, you need to just make a few changes to how you deal with your diet. By all means, you can still eat pasta and rice, but you have to be careful with the options that you choose.

Take that white rice and swap it for brown rice. Take that white pasta that you love and change it for whole-wheat pasta and nothing else.

There are so many other options when it comes to flour, so if you use it in your cooking, then look for some alternatives and throw out that white flour.

Of course, there is also the issue of you snacking on the wrong things. Think of a vegetable smoothie, rather than a fruit one as that's high in sugar, or stack up on vegetables as part of your meal so that the need for a snack is not so problematic.

By making these few changes, you can expect to see a difference in the amount of belly fat that you will then have around your middle.

In this instance, you should look at trying to have a diet that contains less than 50g of refined carbs per day. Being under this level has been shown to be effective in helping people to lose belly fat thanks to that reduction in conversion into stored sugar.

In fact, a study that was primarily looking at heart health also discovered that those individuals that focused on a wholegrain and unrefined carbs diet had a significant decrease of around 17% compared to those individuals that were eating the wrong carbs.

Step 4

Increase Your Soluble Fiber

Fiber is good for your body in a whole host of ways, but you need to be careful with the type of fiber that you are increasing in your diet.

In this instance, we are dealing with soluble fiber, and we need to explain just why this is so important when you are looking at trying to shed that belly fat.

In all honesty, it is just a clever way of stopping you from eating as much and cutting your calorie intake.

By eating more soluble fiber, it will absorb water in your digestive system and make you feel full faster and for longer. If your stomach is telling your brain that it has had enough, then the hunger switch is turned to off.

It has also been shown in some clinical studies that there may very well be a direct link between the amount of soluble fiber you consume and the amount of belly fat you have then decreasing.

In a study that covered over 1000 adults over a 5-year period, it became apparent that increasing your soluble fiber intake by 10g resulted in a reduction of 3.7% of belly fat. This was then repeated if you increased it by yet another 10g.

Getting to Grips with the Mechanics of Soluble Fiber

This is one of those times where the human body and Mother Nature really show how intelligent they both are with the way in which you can benefit from soluble fiber.

You may be aware that there are two types of fiber, soluble and insoluble. In this instance, the insoluble version is pretty boring and is useless. However, the same cannot be said for the soluble version as that can have a pretty powerful impact on your belly fat issue.

But here's the thing. Fiber cannot be digested by the body in the usual way. It just does not work like that.

However, if you could venture into your digestive tract, then you would come across billions upon billions of bacteria that is known as your gut flora.

These bacteria have to be in good working order and they will digest the fiber leading to an improvement in your health.

However, at the same time, the fiber in the digestive tract will reduce inflammation, and this inflammation is seen as being a major contributing factor to weight gain, and guess where that weight gain tends to be focused? Your middle.

Viscose soluble fiber will form an almost gel like substance in your belly. This idea of gel in your stomach does sound pretty horrific, but it is more useful than you think. It forms a gel thanks to its water absorbent properties and as it then takes longer for it to be broken down, it gives you that full feeling longer than insoluble fiber.

Where to Get Soluble Fiber

You could be forgiven for sitting there wondering where on earth you get soluble fiber from as the term may be completely new to you. If that's the case, then it is a lot easier than you may have been expecting. In fact, you are probably already consuming some of it on a daily basis.

For this, you are looking at peas, beans, legumes, oat bran, seeds, nuts, and barley. There are also some fruits and vegetables that also contain a certain amount of soluble fiber, but the items listed above are certainly the best option.

Your Steps to Follow

Making this change to your diet is very easy. You simply need to incorporate the food groups mentioned above and eliminate the bad items. There is nothing else to it.

Oh, you do have to be careful with the quantities, but as we are talking about soluble fiber, this is less of an issue than you may have been expecting. Of course, you need to include the various other changes to your diet if you wish to succeed in losing that belly fat.

I hope that you are enjoying this book so far, and if you could spare 30 seconds, I would greatly appreciate you leaving a review on Amazon.com.

Step 5

Cut Back on the Alcohol Consumption

We aren't saying that everyone should stop drinking alcohol, but there is a very real need for you to look at cutting back on how much you consume on a regular basis.

Numerous studies have shown that an increase in the amount of alcohol you consume has a direct correlation with an increase in belly fat, as well as other health problems. This increase is due to the number of calories and level of sugar that is in alcohol, something which is often surprising to people.

Not only that, but it has been proven that alcohol has the ability to slow down the fat burning process in the body. This slowing down will be a huge problem simply because the first place where the body is going to store that fat that's not being burnt off is going to be in your belly area.

Yet another study indicated that those individuals that consumed two or more alcoholic drinks per day on average had an 80% higher chance of an increase in belly fat than those that either drank less alcohol or none at all.

When you look at statistics and research such as that, then it starts to become difficult to ignore the conclusions that you then have to draw from them.

So, if you want to get rid of that belly fat, then eliminate as much alcohol as possible. It just makes life easier, as well as your body healthier.

Alcohol is Useless Calories

Here is something for the scientists out there, alcohol is often regarded by nutritionists as having empty calories. In short, this means that they are calories that really offer our body nothing apart from making our liver work even harder than it should be doing. But it gets worse.

If you have wine with food, then you are making life even harder for yourself when it comes to the belly fat. Your body is going to take the energy from both the alcohol and carbohydrates and use them for energy as the first port of call.

Now, this might sound good, but it's actually not. As a result of this, the food that you are eating, which tends to be the biggest amount, is then not going to be processed and, as a result, it is then turned into fat which is stored in your body.

So, you are not only making your liver work harder, but you are also actively encouraging your body to put on weight. It's hardly worth it in the end.

Alcohol Affects Hormones

There is also something else going on inside your body when you drink alcohol on a regular basis, and we are not talking about your liver or kidneys which are both already battling.

Alcohol also hampers the production of various hormones in your body. This, in turn, can have a knock-on effect with the way in which your body deals with that belly fat.

In short, it slows down the ability of the body to remove the fat or use it up for energy, so you are then going to have to work even harder than before if you want to stand a chance of shedding that belly fat.

How to Change Things

We could easily sit here and argue that you should eliminate all alcohol and that solves the entire problem, but life isn't always as easy as that. Instead, if you do want to still drink alcohol then there are a few things you can do.

First, don't go and start eating junk food when you are drinking alcohol. That idea that it lines your stomach may very well be true, but just cast your mind back to the point where we said that your body will just turn that food to fat.

Also, there are low-calorie drinks out there, so consider trying to find them as that is also going to make a difference with the calorie count.

Of course, you can also drink water in between alcoholic drinks since that will help to fill you up and it is known to also help people to cut back on the amount of alcohol that they then drink.

There is a reason why you have something called a beer belly.

Take that as absolute truth, so if you continue to drink alcohol, even if you are a binge drinker, then you are just making life so much harder for yourself when it comes to trying to get rid of that belly fat.

Step 6

Boost the Protein

Yes, this is another dietary aspect, but it is one that is very important for your potential success of shedding that belly fat.

Protein plays a major role in weight control. By increasing the level of protein that you are consuming, it results in your body releasing a hormone known as PYY. This hormone is key as it is the hormone that tells your body it is full, so you will then stop eating as you feel that your stomach just cannot take any more food.

Of course, this will then reduce the number of calories that you consume on a daily basis due to that full feeling, and that can only be a good thing for that belly fat.

But there is more to it than that.

You need protein to help with the lean muscle mass, which is important when you are looking at trying to lose any weight or fat on your body. Without this, your body is going to try to use some of the muscle for fuel, when in actual fact you want it to focus on the abdominal fat so that it can vanish from sight.

Now, why should you focus primarily on a high protein diet? Well, if we can go back to scientific research, then what we see is that those individuals that adopt a high protein diet have significantly lower levels of abdominal fat than those on a low protein diet.

In this instance, the argument is that you need to change the protein levels to stop more belly fat being put on or else you will be entering into this vicious cycle that you can never get out of.

Protein Adding Fat is a Myth

This is a point that we need to address as some people believe that increasing your amount of protein will only ever lead to you putting on some additional fat. However, this is a myth.

In fact, if you cut your calories and cut your protein at the same time, then your body is going to use up muscle mass as fuel leading to all kinds of issues.

Instead, nutritional studies have shown that protein helps you to maintain that fat burning muscle, so by increasing your muscle mass, it actually means that the opposite happens to what people expect.

How cool is that?

How Much Do You Eat?

So, you are getting the idea of the role that protein is able to play when it comes to you losing belly fat, but this does depend on you understanding how much of it you need to eat to ultimately get the kind of effects that you were hoping for.

Now, there is no set rule that will work for everyone, but we can offer some guidance just to help you along your way.

For the average adult that does not really workout, but is still looking at losing weight by cutting calories, there is a need for you to consume roughly 1g of protein for every pound of body weight that you have.

You can go as low as 0.8g, but at this moment mixed in with your lack of movement, you really should not go above that 1g figure.

These figures will help you to not only put on some muscle, and prevent muscle loss, but your body is getting enough protein to kick in the fat-burning muscles that then help with the loss of fat in your body.

If you are an adult female who is looking at toning up and losing fat around the middle, then the amount of protein that you should be consuming on a daily basis is higher than that of the individual who is sitting doing nothing much at all.

In this instance, you are looking at trying to consume anywhere between 1g and 1.2g of protein for every pound you weigh. You can go slightly above that top figure, but then you need to work that bit harder to make sure that there are no issues that then develop.

Finally, for an adult male, the figure is higher still thanks to the biological differences between the two sexes.

For this, you are looking at a figure of anywhere between 1g and 1.5g, although the upper end of that figure is actually the preferred amount.

Get to grips with the concept of protein and increase it in your diet as you are more than likely not meeting the minimum requirements for what you are trying to do, which is to remove that belly fat.

Once again, thank you for reading this book, and I hope you're getting a lot of valuable information. I would greatly appreciate it if you could take 30 seconds to leave me a review for this book on Amazon.com.

Enjoying this book?

Check out my other best sellers!

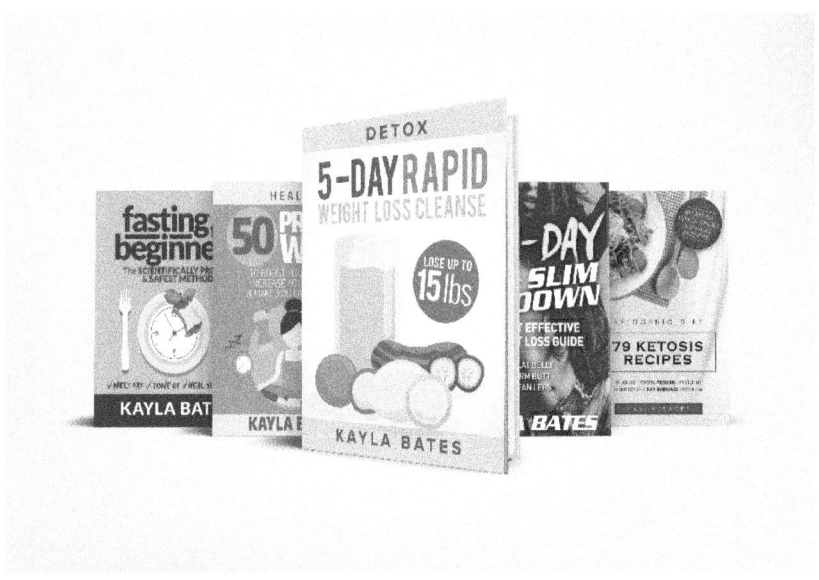

Get your next book on sale here:

TopFitnessAdvice.com/go/Kayla

Step 7

Look at Your Stress Levels

We hinted at this earlier on in the book, but now is the time to look more closely at the role that stress can play in helping you to lose that belly fat.

Aside from your diet, there is one other thing that is a major contributor to the amount of fat that you store around your belly, cortisol.

Now, if you have never heard of cortisol, then it is the hormone that our body releases when we are stressed.

At these times, your body is also going to produce additional hormones including epinephrine and that too will add to the belly fat that you then have to fight to remove from your body.

This hormone is produced in the adrenal glands, and it is directly related to the 'fight or flight' complex that will be familiar to all of us when we are stressed, anxious or afraid.

However, too much stress is bad for not only your health in general, but also your levels of belly fat.

If your cortisol levels are increased, especially for an extended period of time, then it increases your appetite. This increase is directly linked to the body wanting something to give it increased energy for the fight or flight response.

However, we end up storing it, and obviously our body is going to store it in and around your middle.

In other words, stress triggers an automatic response in your body to increase the storage of abdominal fat to be used at a later date.

But it gets worse, especially for women that may have a naturally larger waist. In this instance, it has also been identified that women with a larger waist will then produce more cortisol.

This further increase will then push you into a cycle whereby stress adds belly fat, leading to more upset, which produces more cortisol, and so it goes on.

So, there is only one solution in this instance, and that solution is to cut back on your stress levels as quickly as possible.

How Stress Adds Fat

We mentioned cortisol and the role it plays in adding belly fat to the equation, but we can delve into this in a bit more detail.

There is a direct link between cortisol and glucose levels, so your blood sugar levels are affected by stress.

Of course, when those levels are high it just leads to your body being unable to deal with the sugar and fat content like it would do if it was healthy, so you can start to see how stress does then lead to the addition of fat.

Stress Management and Diet in Tandem

Perhaps the key point that we are making here is connected to the way in which you have to combine stress management with your diet if you are to ever hope to move that abdominal fat.

One helps the other, and yet if you are trying to diet and watch what you eat, but are stressed at the same time, then it is actually pretty pointless.

But here is something that is often overlooked by people that are stressed and dealing with handling a diet, and that is the role that certain foods have in producing inflammation in the body.

Inflammation causes stress on the body, so it is in effect an internal stress whereas most people are just concerned with an external stress.

The kind of foods that you need to avoid are those that are low in fiber and high in trans-fats. Also, red meat should not be eaten on a regular basis as that just further compounds the problem.

Dairy products that are classed as being full fat are also an issue and if you are just filling your body with those kinds of foods, then aside from the fat content, the stress will also be a huge problem that your body is going to struggle to deal with.

So, you need to increase the fiber content, and as we have mentioned in other steps you also need to miss out those refined carbohydrates or anything else that is going to have a profound impact on those glucose levels. It really is not worth the hassle and the extra work that you then have to put into moving that belly fat.

How to Reduce Stress to Help Losing Belly Fat

There are various ways in which you can lose stress to help you with ultimately losing belly fat and you are advised to incorporate as many of them as you can in your day to day routine.

For example, if you have never tried yoga or meditation, then now would be a great time to get started. The same goes for tai chi as they are all about calming the mind and just getting that cortisol flow to stop in its tracks.

At the same time, you must identify the various stressors that you have in your life and take steps to counteract them. Learn how to say no to people if they are putting too much pressure on you because that reluctance to let people down is only going to add to your stress, and your belly fat, of course.

There are clearly going to be a whole host of ways in which you can reduce stress, and it is up to you to find the things that work best for you.

After all, you know what relaxes and soothes your mind and body, so make time for those things in amongst changing your diet and doing the correct exercise and your body will then reward you by starting to reduce that stubborn belly fat.

Step 8

Get the Cardio Workouts Started

It's hardly a surprise that some form of exercise has been included here, but we have to be very specific in the type of exercise that we are talking about if you are serious about losing that belly fat. At this moment, we are focusing on aerobic exercise, also known as cardiovascular exercise.

This approach to working out has been shown to be the most effective way to lose that belly fat. The only problem is that it is actually very difficult to do, so tenacity will play an important role if you are to succeed.

Now, it could be argued that even if you are brand new to doing cardio that anything will make a difference, and that is certainly true.

However, don't expect just a few workouts to make a noticeable difference. It just does not work like that.

Just before we go into the kind of workouts that you should be doing to deal with that abdominal fat, we need to stress one thing.

You do not have to work out as if you are entering the Olympic marathon. This is not a competition or a race. It is something that is personal to you, and you need to really listen to your body if you are to avoid running into problems connected to pushing yourself too hard.

How Cardio Workouts Help

It will perhaps be useful for us to look at how cardio workouts help us to lose that belly fat as this can act as a source of inspiration for you to get that motivation going on those tough days.

Cardio is a great way for burning calories. However, you need to combine this with a reduced intake of calories as part of your diet, or you will just be doing the workout and getting very few benefits from it.

When you do cardio, your body needs energy in order to keep itself going. It will turn to fat stores as its fuel, and it has been shown that one of the areas that it uses as a fat store is your abdomen.

This approach will be hard work, but it has been shown time and time again to be a vital part in the entire process of losing visceral fat, so the scientific proof is there.

The Exercise or the Intensity?

Now, it is perfectly understandable if you are sitting there wondering what exercise is best for you to really hit that belly fat hard. Well, the truth is that it is less to do with the actual form of exercise and more to do with the intensity of the workout.

It has been shown in sports studies that high intensity cardio workouts, even if they involve interval training, are the most effective way of tackling and reducing belly fat as well as improving your overall fitness.

In the main study, they looked at a number of mature individuals who worked out with their heart rate up by 75% and burned around 1000 calories per week due to working out. What it showed was that, after 12 weeks, there was a noticeable difference in the amount of visceral fat that was measured in their body.

However, if the intensity meant that their heart rate was even at just 50%, there was a drop in the amount of visceral fat that they were able to lose.

In other words, the intensity is indeed vital so pushing yourself that bit harder, even for a shorter period of time, will prove to be far more beneficial.

Working that High-Intensity Cardio

So, when we are talking about high-intensity cardio, what do we actually mean?

There are a few options out there, and you should find it quite easy to get something that fits in with your own personal fitness levels.

Remember, it is the intensity that will help you to lose that belly fat, so the way in which you perhaps perform certain actions is less important than you were perhaps aware.

Here is an example. With this, you can easily swap the exercise bike for the treadmill or rowing machine as they all do the same thing to your body and heart rate.

First, you need to always warm up, and do so at a nice easy pace as this is more about getting the heart rate increased slowly and also warming up the muscles. This should last for between five to ten minutes as by then things should be moving well and your body is prepared for a more intense bout of exercise.

After this, it is time to start pushing yourself and really getting that heart rate up to around 75% of your maximum heart rate.

If possible, which means if your general fitness levels allow it, you should be aiming for working out at this rate for a minimum of 20 minutes.

In fact, that should be your first goal, but then you can go longer if you are fit enough and are not going to be putting your body under too much stress.

Of course, there is always a need for you to cool down after this, which means gradually slowing things down to a leisurely speed for another 5 minutes or so as this just helps everything in your body to settle down in a more natural way and stop potential injuries.

How Much Belly Fat Will You Lose?

This is the million-dollar question, but it is also the hardest question to answer. To be honest, it is impossible to answer as there are so many decisive factors that need to be taken into account.

Instead, what we can do is look at the average for a 30-minute-long high intensity routine and the number of calories that you will typically burn. This will, in turn, allow you to work out the dietary aspect and the calorie count part.

If we say that we are talking about someone who weighs 155 pounds, then you are looking at burning some 400 calories on a stationary bike and almost the same when you are running for 30 minutes at a speed of 6 mph.

Even step aerobics will be burning off approximately 370 calories and then a stair stepper still burns off 220 calories, which is still better than nothing.

Of course, that does not really allow us to convert it into a percentage of belly fat, but it could easily be argued that anything is better than nothing.

However, you need to work out on a regular basis to get the benefit from it, and clearly just doing these high intensity cardio workouts are not the only thing that you need to do to get rid of that belly fat.

Indeed, even with exercise there is one other area that you should focus on and that is trying to incorporate lifting weights into your routine, although with that there are also certain things that you should focus on if you really want to deal with your belly fat once and for all.

Others who are considering purchasing this book would love to know what you think. If you could spare a few seconds, they would greatly appreciate reading an honest review from you. Simply visit the page on Amazon.com.

Step 9

Lift Weights in Your Routine

Sticking with the workout aspect, a lot of people will hit the gym and pump some iron, and while this does indeed make a difference, there is a very real need to keep close control over what you lift and how often.

The other important thing is that this should be done in tandem with your cardio workout. A study that focused on teenagers that were overweight showed that incorporating both into your workout routines will lead to the greatest decrease in percentage of visceral fat, and with that it means the belly fat is going to vanish.

The problem here is that people think that lifting weights leads to building muscle, and that muscle is heavy. However, even though that is indeed true, we need to look past that and focus on the way in which it can really benefit your abdomen and the distribution of that visceral fat.

How it Helps

Lifting weights clearly helps you to build muscle mass, and this is important for the sake of burning off fat.

If you increase your muscle mass, then what happens is you improve the ability of your body to burn calories while at rest, so you do actually benefit from this when tackling that belly fat issue.

The reason for this is simply because your muscles need more energy than fat in order to maintain themselves at their level. Plus, you are moving them in some way throughout the entire day, so that clearly uses up more energy, so your body looks at those fat stores to help.

But there is more to it than this, and it is all to do with your age and metabolic rate.

As you get older, you lose muscle mass and your metabolism slows down naturally. That is why we find it harder to avoid putting on weight as we get older.

Weight training has been shown in studies to be an effective tool in fighting back against that drop in your metabolic rate, so your body will then work against that excess belly fat appearing in the first place.

Pairing Lifting Weights with Cardio

In step 8, we spoke about the importance of high-intensity cardio for losing that belly fat, but when you combine it with lifting weights, then you are going to really hit that fat hard, and see better results in a shorter period of time.

What the studies have shown is that you need to do high intensity cardio workouts as well as high intensity resistance training to ultimately lose the most belly fat in the shortest period of time.

At first, you should be looking at trying to do at least two weight training sessions per week, and you must focus on the key muscle groups and build them on a regular basis. This means you must work the arms, back, chest, shoulders, abdomen, legs, and hips.

By working them, you will notice that you lose fat over your entire body, and as a result it also has an impact on your abdomen with an obvious reduction being seen in a few weeks.

Yes, a few weeks as there is no quick answer to this, so you have to be prepared to really work at it if you are serious about getting results.

How to Proceed

If you are unsure about lifting weights or even the correct exercises to do, then consider getting an assessment from a personal trainer. They can offer you the correct advice and also the way to gradually build the weights you lift followed by the increase in your muscle mass.

Of course, you need to start out relatively low both in weight as well as repetitions.

However, there is a need for you to increase the intensity, and with the weight you should be looking at using something that feels heavy once you have done between eight to twelve repetitions.

This number of repetitions equals one set. You should begin by doing one set and try to work it up to three sets before you then increase the weight further.

There is no way we can turn around and say how much belly fat you will lose due to lifting weights, but as we have said elsewhere any difference will be better than you sitting there and doing nothing about it.

Remember, it is more to do with muscle mass and the way in which it boosts your metabolism and ability to burn fat even while at rest that is important.

So, drop that idea that lifting weights will do nothing. It's wrong and you are doing yourself a real injustice by not incorporating some high resistance level weight training in your routine.

Step 10

Get into a Better Routine

In this instance, what we are specifically talking about is getting into a better life routine in general. This means so much more than just watching what you eat or drink. It also means making sure that you get enough sleep and rest.

Now, you might be thinking that rest means being inactive, and surely that is causing part of the problem?

Well, not exactly.

Instead, what we are talking about is primarily the number of hours you spend getting quality sleep at night.

This all comes from sleep studies and how they relate to our ability to either lose weight or put it on. What it shows is that if you continually have inadequate sleep, then your body is going to slow down your metabolism and you will then start to put on weight.

Now, guess where on your body that weight is going to be applied? That's right, around your middle.

The exact reason as to why it does this is not that important. What is important for you is the understanding that you need to get at least 7 hours of sleep a night to help you get rid of that belly fat.

Once again, this can be seen as a preventative measure, and the plan here is that these small changes to your routine and general quality of life will stop your body from adding on more belly fat at any given opportunity.

If you stop your body from resorting to this, then it makes sense that it is then easier for you to get rid of the belly fat that is already there. Your body can focus on that fat rather than trying to deal with the new layers that are appearing.

More on Tackling Sleep Issues

If we are suffering from sleep issues whereby we are forcing ourselves into a routine where we are not getting an ample number of hours, then we have a tendency to do some rather distinct things to keep us going.

Primarily, we will drink coffee, or energy drinks and clearly this is going to send our blood sugar levels rising, and as we know from other chapters, this adds to belly fat production and storage.

It's almost as if we are overtaken by our desire or need to stay awake that we forget about what kind of fuel we are putting into our bodies.

The difficulty is that, when we are tired, our brain starts to work a bit differently. We have a lessening of our impulse control and the possibilities of us making some bad decisions are only going to be increased. That is what then leads to us having those snacks and food cravings are horrific at this moment in time.

As our impulse control is impaired, it does then mean we are more likely to give in and eat or drink something that we would have avoided had we been well rested.

At the same time, we not only have a tendency to eat something that has a higher number of carbs, but we also eat larger portions, so that calorie count is going to be destroyed in an instant.

How to Repair it

The answer is easy, get somewhere between 7 and 9 hours of sleep every single night. The benefits are clear for all to see. It reduces your stress levels – so you lose belly fat that way – and you make better decisions when it comes to eating the correct things at the correct time.

Also, if your body is able to fire on all cylinders due to having had enough sleep, it also means that you are going to burn calories better than you would if your body and mind were tired. Clearly, this can only be a good thing for losing that belly fat.

In other words, an unsettled night on a regular basis will be bad news for you and your quest to lose that belly fat. Your body as a whole slows down and is unable to cope satisfactorily with the stresses of day to day life.

Other Aspects of a Good Routine that Helps

Clearly there will be more to the routine than just sleeping enough during the night as even something as simple as eating at regular intervals makes a difference to your belly fat issue. Too often, we are rushed into eating or just grab something when we can, and yet that is the wrong thing to do.

If your body is unaware of when it can expect the next intake of food, then it switches into starvation mode. This is something that harks back to when food could be scarce and the body developed a method to combat this.

What happens in starvation mode is the body will store any food as fat so it can then be used as energy later on. This helps to act as sustenance and provide you the energy to do the things you need to do in order to then get more food.

Because of this, your body will store fat in various areas, and it is known that the primary area is your abdomen. Erratic eating is just as bad for visceral fat as what you eat, and if you combine both bad habits together, then you have a major problem on your hands.

I hope you have learned something from this book so far and would greatly appreciate it if you could leave an honest review on Amazon.com.

Step 11

Watch What You Drink

We mentioned alcohol in an earlier step, but this time we are looking at something slightly different.

The difficulty for most people is that they have this wrong impression of what is good for your health and losing belly fat, and what is bad. This leads to all kinds of mistakes, and then we find ourselves wondering just why exactly we are not making the progress that we hoped for.

People will often switch to what they believe to be a healthy way of eating. Included in this will be fruit juice. People are drawn into the belief that it's only fruit juice, and so it is going to be good for us, and from a vitamins and minerals point of view, this is true.

However, there is one massive problem, and it is a problem that is further exacerbating the issue of belly fat, natural sugars.

No matter the fruit juice that you are drinking, there will be high concentrates of fructose, a naturally occurring sugar that appears in fruit.

Your body will, of course, use this for energy and as we have explored in previous steps, it is going to keep that sugar stored as fat via glucose for whenever it is required in the future.

In other words, if you consume considerable quantities of fruit juice, then you will see an increase in the level of belly fat rather than a decrease.

If you are sitting there thinking that the sugar in fruit juice surely can't be that bad, then think of this one thing. It has been shown that the levels of sugar in pure orange juice, apple juice, or whatever tends to be equal to the sugar that appears in a can of soda.

At times, it can actually be higher, and yet people think that they are doing a good thing by their body.

This just shows how easy it is to make a mistake with this kind of thing, but it will then often lead to people wondering what exactly they can then drink that then doesn't lead to these kinds of issues.

There are several options that are available to you. First, you can increase the amount of water that you drink and this tends to be one of the best things that you can do.

Of course, water is going to have no sugar or calories, so there is nothing to worry about from that perspective.

However, it also makes you feel full and brings your appetite to a halt, and clearly this is also going to be a positive.

Step 12

Keep Track of Things

The 12th and final step is more important than you realize.

Anybody that has tried to lose some weight will be able to testify that you get to this point where you feel as if you are making no progress whatsoever. You look at yourself in the mirror and you see absolutely no difference.

It is depressing, and you feel like giving up. That is the mistake that most people make. They feel as if they are a failure when, in actual fact, it doesn't have to be true at all.

The key here is to make sure that you do indeed keep track of things. Without this, you can easily trick yourself into believing that there is no difference when, in actual fact, more is happening than you realize.

How annoyed would you be if you found out that you quit when you were actually doing better than you thought? This alone is enough to make you feel depressed and to kick start your body into adding more belly fat.

What we recommend in this instance is going ahead and downloading an app that can make life easier for you. This does mean you are able to keep a note of how you are progressing with you at all times, something that just makes life that little bit easier.

There are several available, and this is undoubtedly something that you want to get into the habit of doing because of the way in which it can boost your confidence and inspire you to keep on going.

Look at it from this perspective. If you believed that you were getting nowhere; how likely are you going to be to then just give up? The chances are that the odds will be very high.

Turn things around for a moment, and imagine how you would feel if you thought you were getting nowhere, but then you looked at your track record and saw that you have still made progress of some kind, even if that is small.

Do you feel that your chances of quitting would increase or decrease? Clearly, they would decrease as you would understand that things had just slowed down somewhat. You wouldn't feel so disheartened by it all that's for sure.

Make notes of what you are eating, the way you are eating, when, and also the kind of exercise you are doing. Take measurements and weigh yourself because you are going to lose weight all over your body as a result of taking these steps to combat that belly fat.

However, don't allow yourself to be drawn into becoming obsessed with the figures. That in itself is not helpful. Just make sure that it is part of your routine, and you will be more likely to go ahead and actually reach those goals.

Don't forget to share your thoughts on this book by leaving a review on Amazon.com. It takes just a few seconds.

Conclusion

So, there you have it, 12 different steps that you should really seriously think about including in your plan to tackle your belly fat issue.

The only additional thing that we should mention is that there is no guarantee of success. It all depends on your willingness to put in the effort.

Belly fat is rightfully seen as being the hardest fat to lose.

However, just because it is hard does not mean that it is impossible. Too many people are defeated before they can even begin. They fall into that trap of believing that they are just not going to manage to do it no matter how much effort they through at it all, or how much they alter their diet.

If you are of that frame of mind, then stop it right now. You are defeating yourself and making it impossible to lose that belly fat all because of what is in your mind.

Losing belly fat requires dedication and a willingness to push yourself both with what you put into your body, and the way you exercise.

It takes work, but it is work that can ultimately pay off for you. It just takes time, so if you are the impatient kind, then all we can say is good luck to you because the near future is going to prove to be rather tough.

Make changes to the way you approach life. Make changes to what you eat and how you exercise.

Losing that belly fat will then become a by-product, and considering the way in which it can become important for your overall health, this is something that is worth doing.

Are You ALWAYS Hungry When You Try to Lose Weight?

Discover How to STOP Starving Yourself & Lose Weight FASTER By Eating MORE Food!

For this month only, you can get Kayla's best-selling & most popular book absolutely free – *The Ultimate Guide to Healthy Eating & Losing Weight Without Starving Yourself!*

Get Your FREE Copy Here:
TopFitnessAdvice.com/Book

Discover how you can **start eating MORE food** and see weight loss results faster than ever before. Learn about the 10 most powerful fat-burning foods and how they boost the rate that your body burns fat. And last but not least, finally put an end to your emotional or "bored" eating habits. With this book, readers were able to significantly improve their weight loss results. So, it's highly recommended that you get this book, especially while it's free!

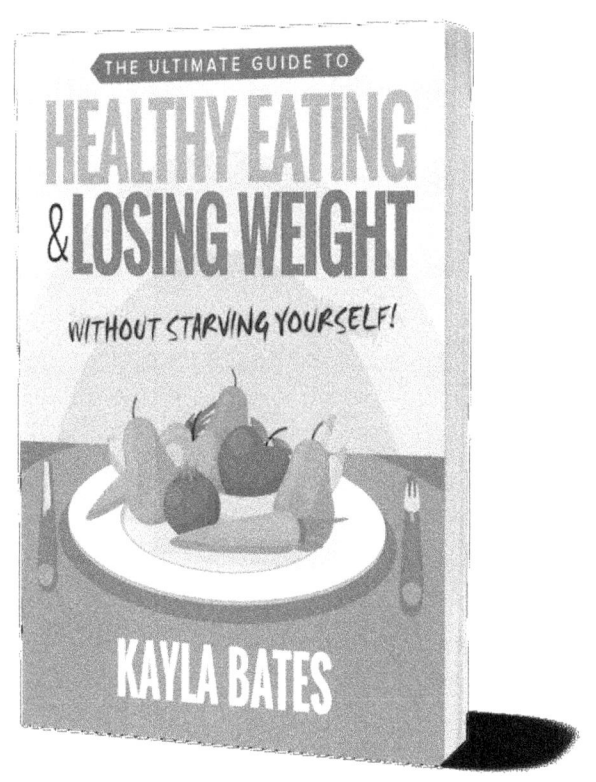

Get Your FREE Copy Here:

TopFitnessAdvice.com/Book

30 Bonus Food Tips

As food and what you eat plays such a huge role in this entire thing, we thought it would be fun to include some 30 bonus recipes to get your mind thinking as to what is possible with food.

Now, you don't need to be some kind of chef to produce things along these lines, but they are all deemed to be good for helping to fight against belly fat while still providing you with all of the nutrition that you need.

1. Kale Salad with Quinoa and Strawberries

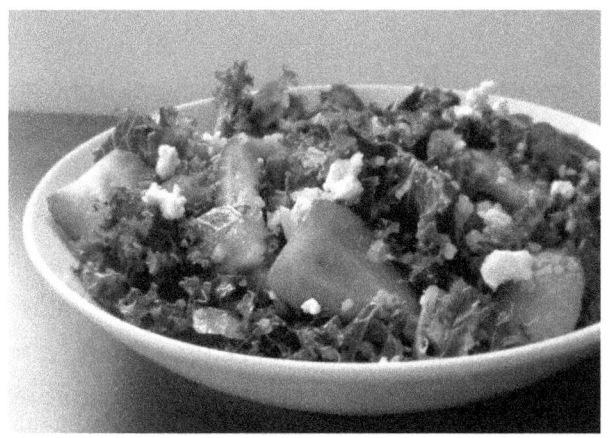

This is seen as being a breakfast, and the potential combination of kale and strawberries may sound strange to most people. However, throw in the quinoa and some seeds, what you get is a balanced and nutritious breakfast that should set you up perfectly for the rest of the day.

2. Smoothies

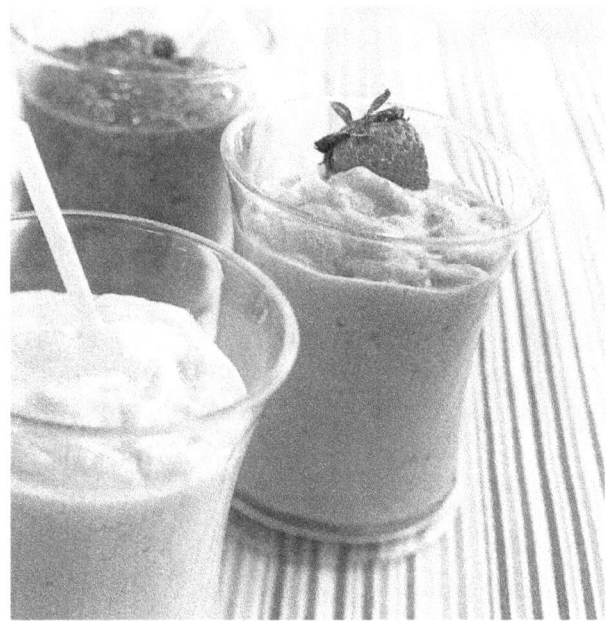

Smoothies are amazing things, but you need to be careful with fruit smoothies because of the sugar content that is in them. To be honest, for the morning it might be better for you to stick with one that is primarily vegetables.

You can throw in an apple or some fruit juice to add a touch of sweetness, but a combination of kale, spinach, cucumber, ginger, parsley, cayenne pepper, orange juice, and lemon juice can be a great way to get a boost of nutrients first thing in the morning.

3. Pancakes with Walnuts and Honey

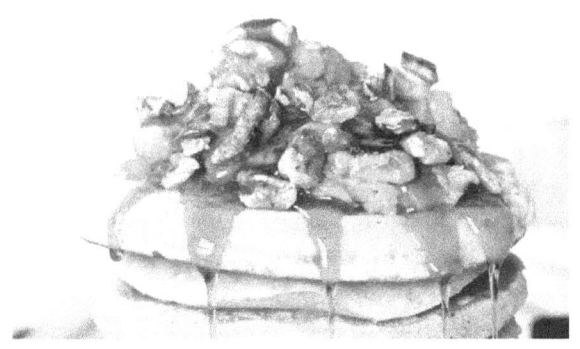

We know that honey is high in sugar, but just a small amount can go a long way. The walnuts are good for your belly fat as they have Omega 3, and if you are concerned about the pancakes, then use gluten free ingredients.

Not only are they filling, but they are also going to be easy for your digestion to deal with. Make things different by throwing in some chopped up banana into the pancake mix.

4. Eggs Florentine with Pesto

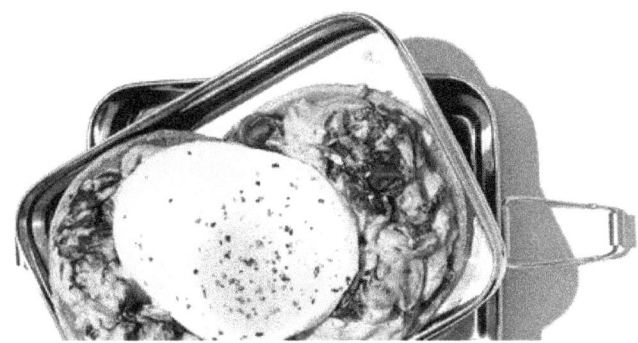

Eggs are good for you and this recipe is yet another amazing breakfast that helps in that fight against belly fat. Get some spinach, eggs, Greek yogurt, some pesto and some English muffins that are toasted.

Blanch the spinach, mix the yogurt and pesto together, and then cook your eggs. Drizzle in some olive oil and then use the half muffin as the base to pile everything onto.

5. Granola

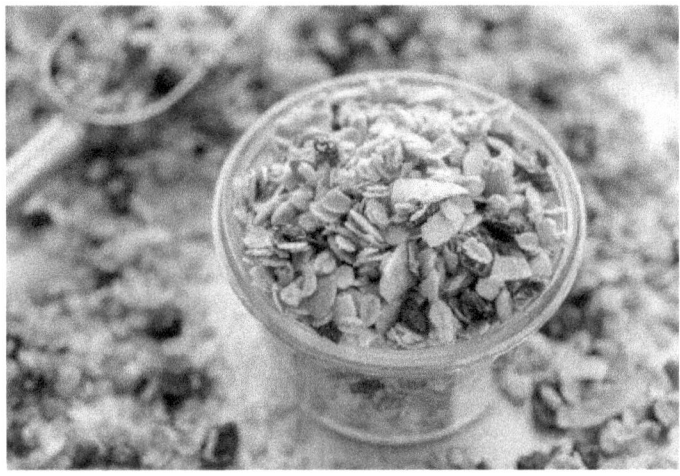

Making your own granola at home is easy. Buy some oats, a mix of different seeds, and some dried fruit of your choice. Mix things together in a bowl and add in a mixture of honey and oil to coat everything.

Spread it on a baking tray and put it in the oven until it is golden brown. Allow it to cool and you have a healthy breakfast.

6. Lettuce Sandwich

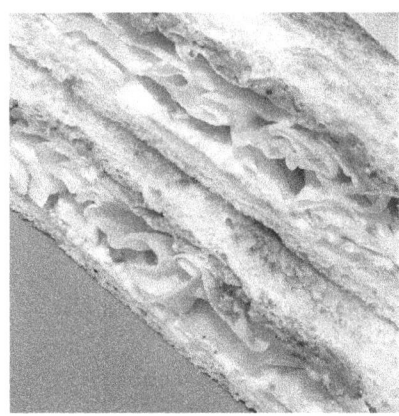

This may very well sound strange, but using lettuce leaves in place of bread can still give you an amazing sandwich. Add in any fillings that you want, but feel so much better about it since you don't have to worry about the bad effects of the bread that you would have otherwise been eating.

7. Tangerine and Beet Salad with Roasted Pistachios

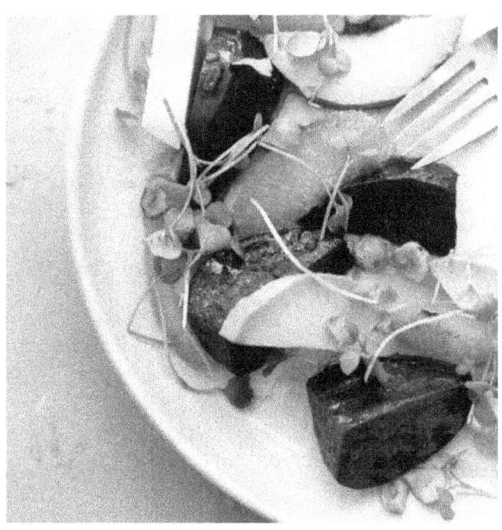

Packed full of flavor and healthy goodness, you just need to roast the beets, including the greens, roast some pistachios, throw in feta and some steamed kale followed by segments of tangerine. It gives you a balanced meal that is perfect for your belly. Consider adding in some chicken as well.

8. Mushroom and Barley Risotto

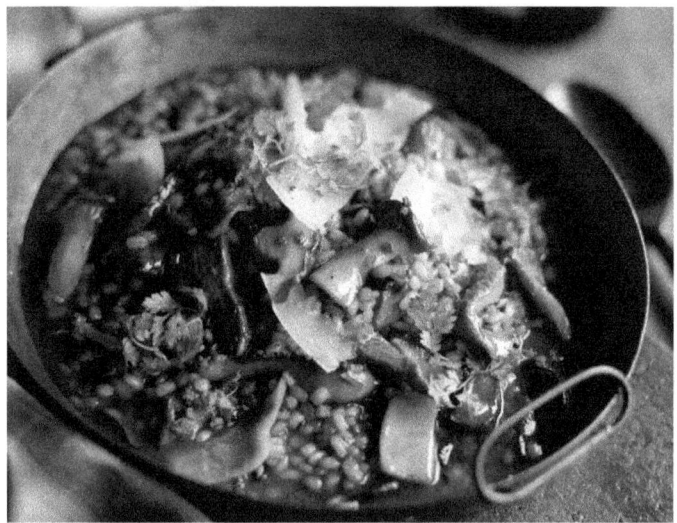

With this, it's best if you can get wild mushrooms but any kind will do. Also, the barley is high in fiber which is always a good thing for your belly as it will make you feel full for longer.

Just gently fry the mushrooms, boil the barley just as you would if making the rice version of risotto, and throw in some rocket as well to add a touch of green to it all.

9. Pepper Salad

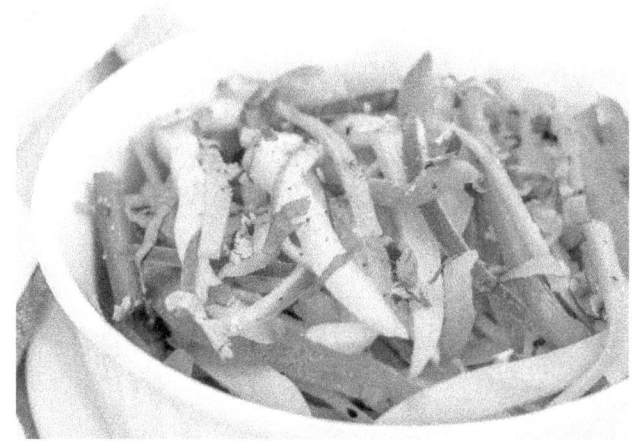

This one has an Italian side to it, so it's packed full of rich colors and nutrients. Get a variety of peppers and gently roast them. Throw in a vinegar dressing along with some seeds and barley and use it as an accompaniment to chicken to allow you to get that hit of protein that you really need in your diet to help combat that belly fat.

10. Rice and Lentil Salad

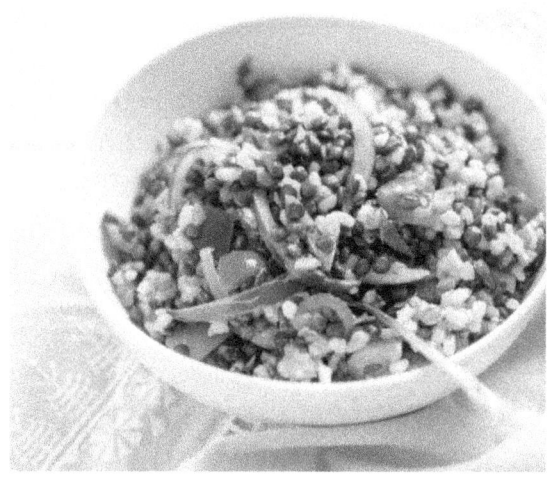

The mixture of rice and lentils gives a good combination and provides you with a lot of protein. To add some spark to it, you should use some vinegar, mustard, and paprika so it has a bit of a kick. Simply cook the individual parts as normal and then combine them along with the dressing for a healthy and nutritious meal.

11. Fettuccine with Brussels Sprouts and Mushrooms

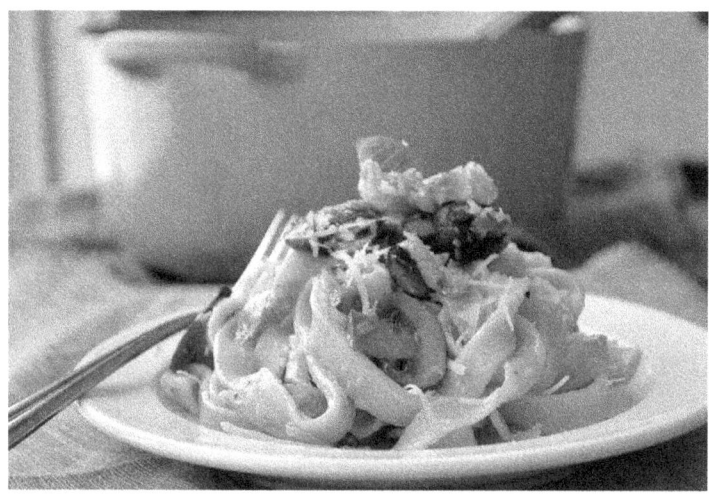

For this, you should use whole-wheat Fettuccine and look at lactose free cream as the sauce. Slice mushrooms and brussels sprouts and quickly fry them. Use some of the juice from the mushrooms to add flavor to the sauce and add the cream and stir it through. Once it has come to the boil and warmed, add to the pasta.

12. Protein Powder Drinks

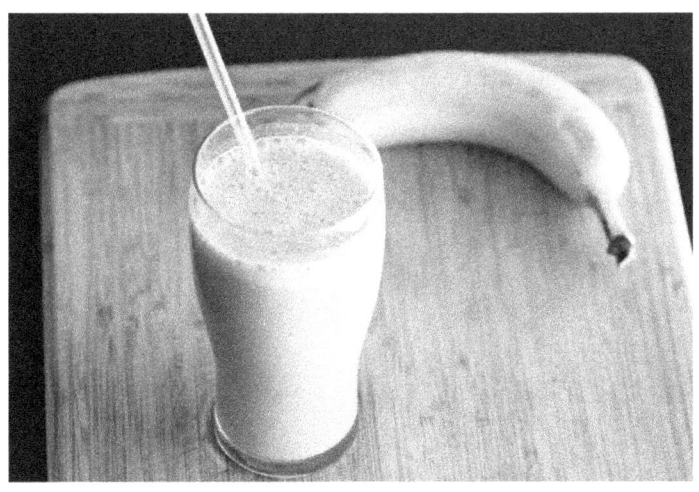

Remember how we said protein was important to lose belly fat? Well, if you are eating primarily salads and worried you are not getting enough, then using a quality protein powder in a drink is a good alternative.

Choose the flavor, make the drink, and it will not only make you feel full, but also help you in your fight.

13. Red Pepper Corn Muffin

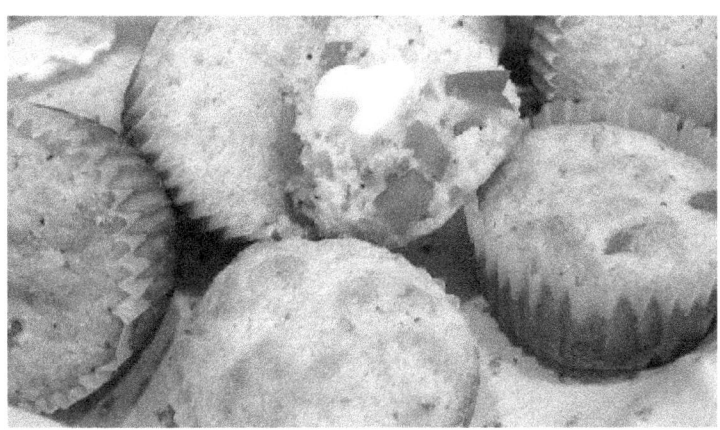

If you want something as a treat, then consider using gluten free options as you make a red pepper corn muffin.

Using corn flour, scallions, peppers, salt, and pepper along with a traditional muffin recipe, you get a breakfast snack or something for a break that is still not going to include too much fat that will then head to your belly.

14. Roast Beef Panini

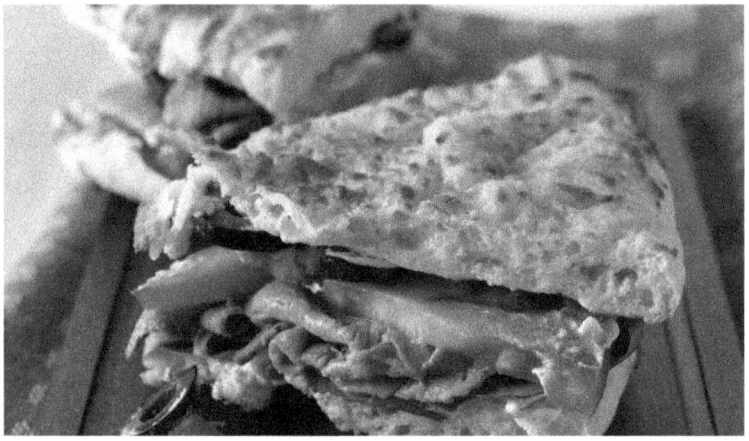

For this, whole-wheat bread can be used, but it is the fillings that are the important part.

You are looking at roast beef, using avocado instead of mayo, along with various salad items to create something that is not only tasty, but full of fat busting nutrients and vitamins. Use olive oil as the spread on the bread and consider adding some mustard to help things along.

15. Moroccan Chicken with Olives

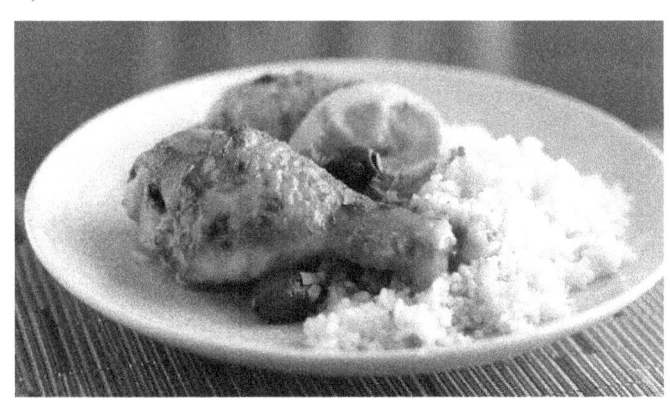

This is one for the slow cooker. Get some chicken broth with reduced salt and add to the slow cooker. Throw in the chicken along with peppers with cumin, pepper, and oil and mix together. Also add in some tomatoes, carrots, olives and garlic and leave it for 3 hours on a high heat. If you want it spicier, then use hotter peppers.

16. Chicken Piccata

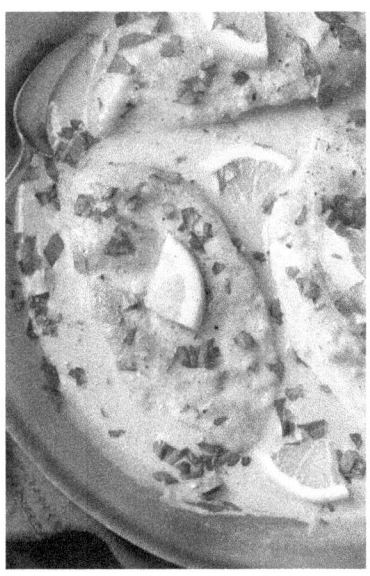

This is an Italian recipe and all you need is some chicken, lemon, capers, parsley, and pepper. Get some alternative to white flour and lightly coat the chicken in it and lightly fry the chicken pieces.

Once it has been browned, throw in the lemon juice, capers and parsley and allow it all to come to the boil. Let it work its magic for 5 minutes before serving.

17. African Chicken Stew

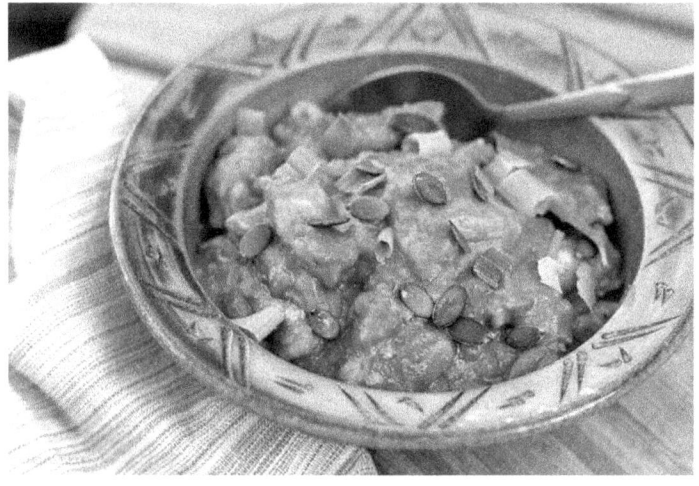

This is another one for the slow cooker and is a combination of chicken, carrots, and potatoes. First, brown the chicken followed by browning some onions, garlic, carrots, and chili pepper for a few minutes.

In a pot, add reduced salt chicken broth before adding all of the ingredients along with some tomato paste and sweet potato and leave it to just simmer away for 5 to 6 hours.

18. Olive and Turkey Pita Sandwich

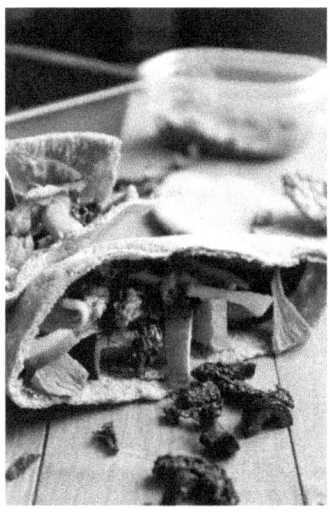

Pita bread is light and should not cause you too many problems. Use it as a wrap and add in your favorite olives, turkey, and salad but add some balsamic vinegar and peppers to add a zing to it and stop it from feeling so boring.

19. Roasted Potatoes with Blue Cheese

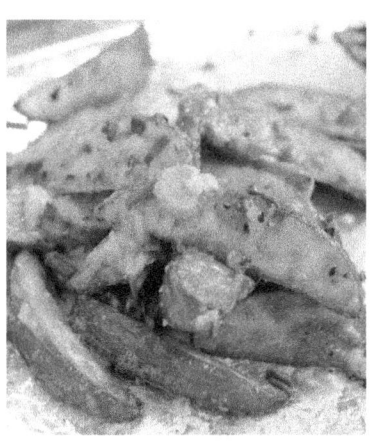

This is better for your belly than fries. Get some baby potatoes and keep the skins on and then halve them. Throw them into a tin and add oil, pepper, and salt. Roast at a high temperature for 30 minutes.

Get another tin and add some walnuts to roast them and then sprinkle in some blue cheese. Add this to the top of the potatoes when they are ready.

20. Steak and Pepper Tacos

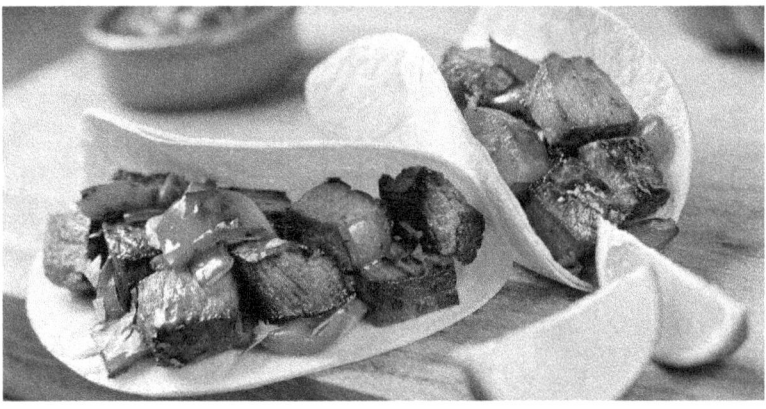

Lean steak, peppers sliced, some limes, salad, low fat cheese grated, and corn tortillas can lead to a wonderful dish that is full of flavor and color at the same time.

You get protein, vitamins, minerals, carbs and a whole lot more, but it is all controlled and will not cause you problems with your belly.

21. Shrimp and Avocado Rice

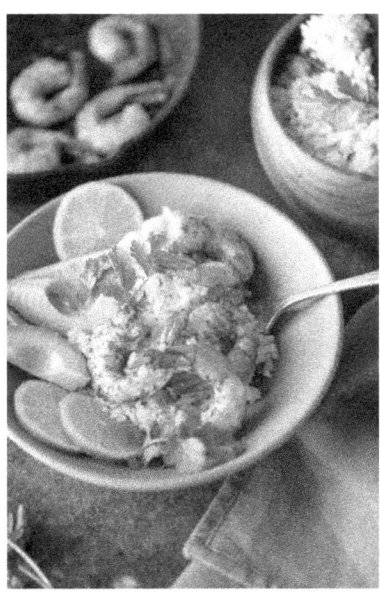

Use brown rice for this dish as it is better for your digestion. Get fresh shrimps and cook them lightly. Throw in some honey and paprika or spice of your choice to give them an extra bite. Use vinegar and soy sauce as a dressing for the rice and then take advantage of the avocado to add some coolness to the dish.

22. Lemon Walnut Chicken

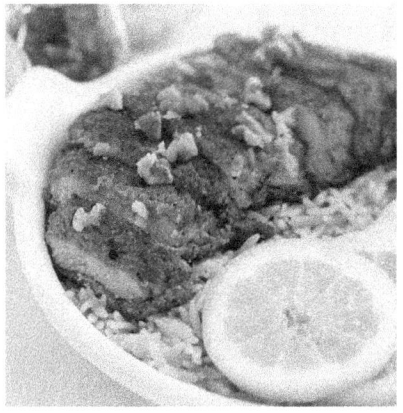

Brown the chicken and then cook slowly in some olive oil. At the same time, chop up parsley and walnuts and grate some lemon zest.

Dice some shallots and throw into a pan to lightly fry them together. This then goes on top of the chicken once it is cooked to add a real bite to your slice of protein.

23. Apple Slices with Cinnamon

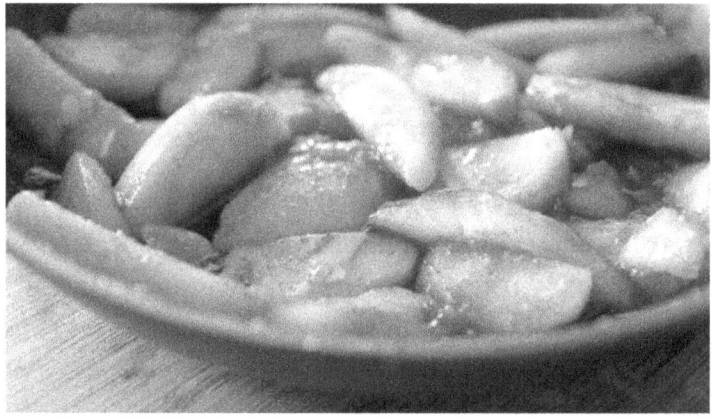

For anybody who is looking for a quick snack, then apple slices with cinnamon is perfect. It's not only low in calories, but it also keeps your blood sugar levels under a certain degree of control stopping issues with insulin and the storage of fat.

By using cinnamon as a replacement for sugar, you are also just giving a healthier side to it.

24. Zoodles with Avocado and Tomato

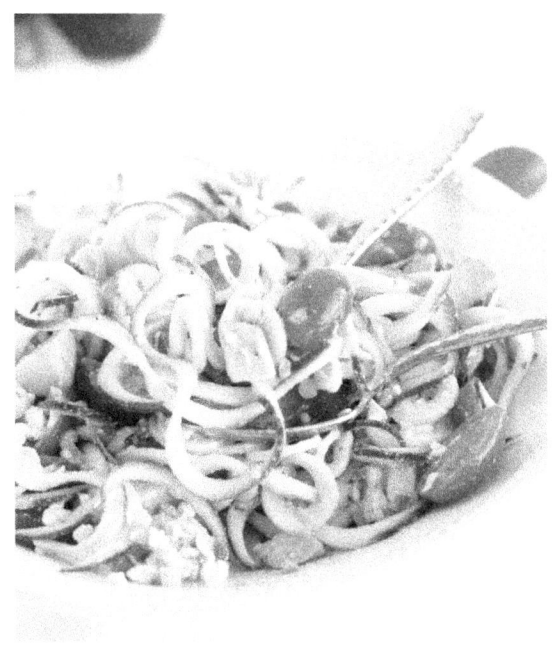

Zoodles are noodles made from zucchini, so you are looking at a low carb option that is not going to cause you the problems often associated with normal noodles.

Cooking them in the same way as noodles, you can then start to add some interest to them by using tomato and mashed up avocado.

This is going to quell your appetite while also providing you with a good source of fiber without being hit by those carbs that lead to belly fat.

25. Romaine and Smoked Salmon Salad

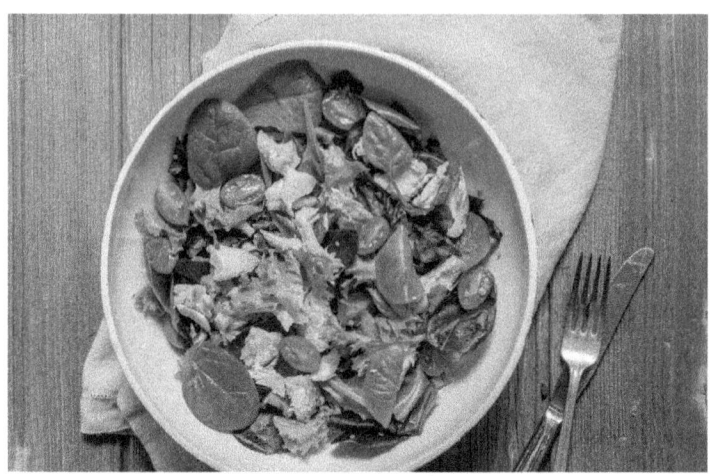

Salmon is high in Omega-3 which is good for your digestion and body in general. Pairing it with Romaine lettuce as the base along with various other raw vegetables, such as radish, carrots and cucumber will help with the fiber issue and there are no additional sugars. Purchase the smoked salmon and you have a very fast and easy meal.

26. Tomato Soup

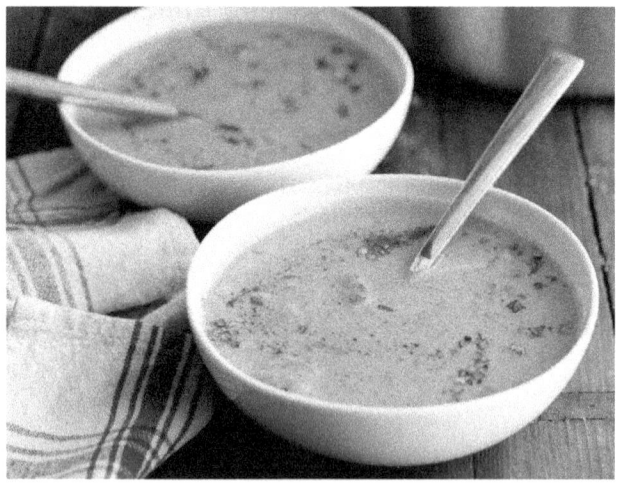

Making your own tomato soup is a wonderful idea. Leave out the cream and use tomatoes, carrots and some celery along with reduced salt vegetable stock. Think about also throwing in some garlic as this also helps with the fat burning aspect. Let it all simmer and then blend to make the soup smooth before serving.

27. Black Bean and Almond Pesto Chicken

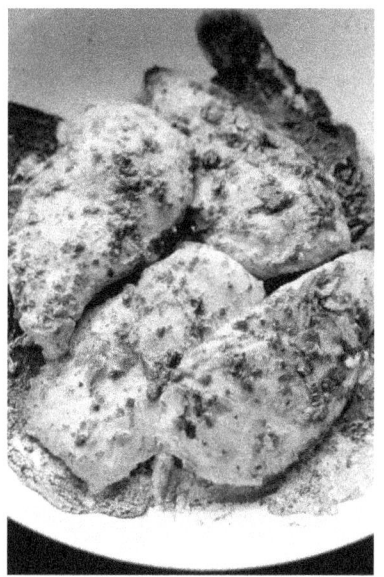

As it has chicken, then you are covering the protein aspect. The beans are high in fiber, which is also good for that belly fat issue. Almonds also help to regulate your blood sugar levels, which does stop the sugar turning to fat. Create a salad with a vinegar dressing, mix the crushed almonds with olive oil and some garlic to make the pesto. Cook the beans as normal, and lightly grill the chicken for a wonderful meal.

28. Lentil Salad with Yellow Tomatoes and Bell Peppers

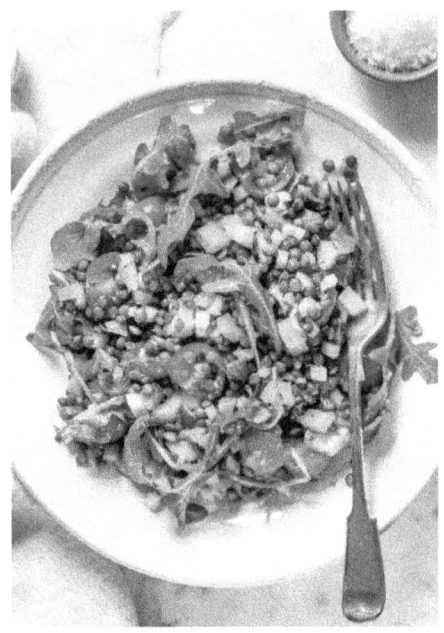

Not only is this colorful, but it is also going to give you a boost of Vitamin C as well as fiber.

It is also very easy to prepare as you simply cook the lentils in some vegetable stock to soften them and then combine with chopped up yellow tomatoes, some bell peppers, onions, lettuce, and add a light vinegar dressing.

29. Chicken Chili

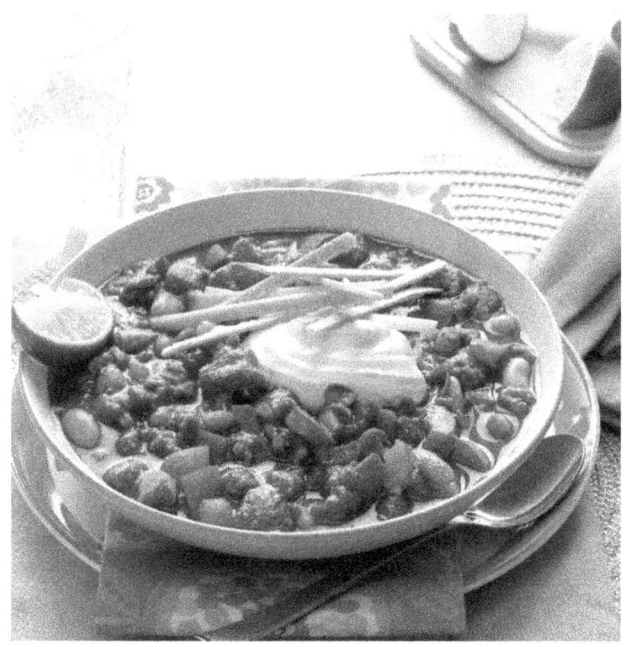

This is for those people that prefer a bit of a kick to their meals as well as making sure that you get your protein.

For this, you need some chicken, canned tomatoes, kidney beans, onions, green peppers, chili powder, and taco seasoning. Place the chicken, onions, peppers and chili powder in a slow cooker for 4 hours.

Once you remove it, cut the chicken into pieces and add the tomatoes, seasoning, and kidney beans to the mix and cook again for another 3 hours.

30. Egg Fried Vegetable Rice

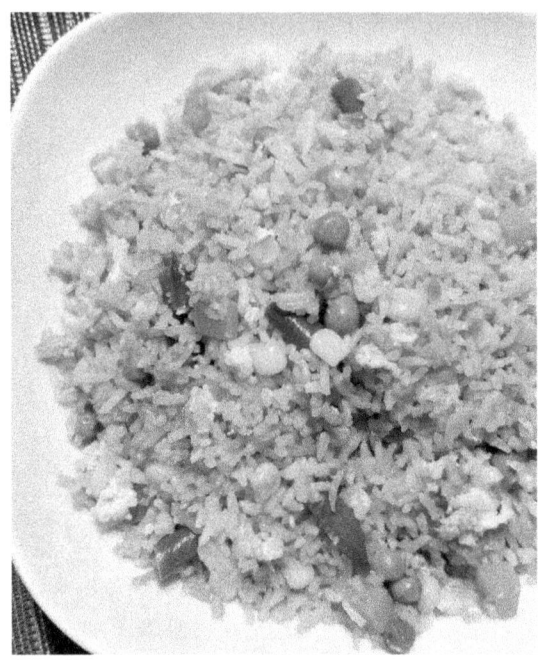

For something from the Orient, you can look at egg fried vegetable rice, just as long as you use brown rice rather than white rice due to the way in which the body processes things differently and the way it stops sugar spikes.

Take some broccoli, baby mushrooms, onions, garlic, and cabbage as your base. Stir fry them in some olive oil and throw in an egg as well. Cook the rice on its own and use some Chinese flavoring to the water. Once it is all cooked, combine the two together.

Final Words

I would like to thank you for purchasing my book and I hope I have been able to help you and educate you on something new.

If you have enjoyed this book and would like to share your positive thoughts, could you please take 30 seconds of your time to go back and give me a review on my Amazon book page.

I greatly appreciate seeing these reviews because it helps me share my hard work.

You can leave me a review on Amazon.com.

Again, thank you and I wish you all the best!

Enjoying this book?

Check out my other best sellers!

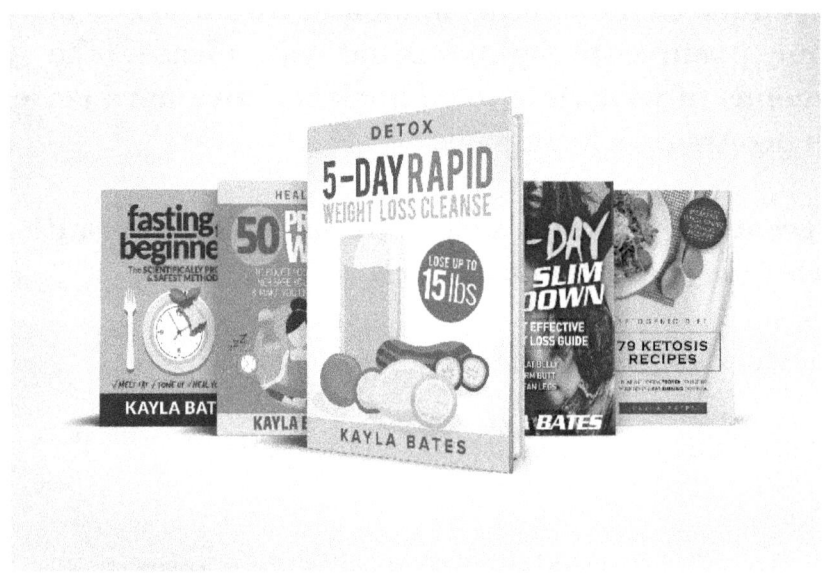

Get your next book on sale here:

TopFitnessAdvice.com/go/Kayla

www.ingramcontent.com/pod-product-compliance
Lightning Source LLC
Chambersburg PA
CBHW031201020426
42333CB00013B/766